No Hogwash
De Stress

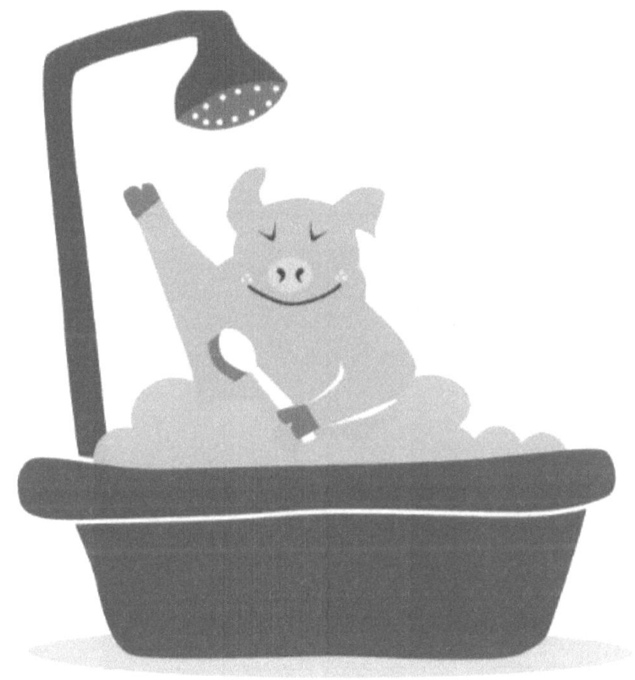

Natural Healing

By: Michael Von Irvin, MBA, BSN, RN

*It is not the strongest of the species that survives, not the most
intelligent that survives. It is the one that is the most adaptable to
change.*
—Charles Darwin

Testimonials
For Michael Von Irvin

Michael
"My pleasure to add a distinguished professional, such as
yourself, to my circle of friends. All the best to you and your
loved ones."
Father of Steve Job's Founder Of Apple Computers
John Jandali

Author • "America's #1 Marketing Wizard" •
• "The Deal Maker" • "Master Negotiator"
A lot of people are saying great things about Mike Von Irvin.

Former New York City Healthcare executive. Former VP of
AlphaCare and Director of Marketing for MLTC Consulting.
Serial Entrepreneur.

Past appearances with Geraldo Rivera, Thomas Mesereau
(Michael Jackson's Attorney), Tracy Morgan, Prince Royce,
Rafael Furcal and many other celebrities, politicians, and sports
stars.

BRANDING—My friend marketing whiz Michael Von Irvin says
branding is pointless without good Copywriting to back it up. I
think he's right.
—David Garfinkel (copywriting legend)

John Fleck
Owner
Wanted to give a shout out to Michael Von Irvin. In one day
his coaching and guidance has made a huge difference in the
direction of my business.

To work with Michael Von Irvin or make comments contact
help@writersprofitguide.com

—Brad Szollose with Michael Von Irvin.
My second business meeting in the city was with businessman, speaker and trainer Michael Von Irvin and his wife Bella.

Some of our clients have included large healthcare plans such as AlphaCare NY - now Magellan Health. Fitango - innovative patient engagement solutions help to reduce costly readmissions and improve outcomes - NY, Special Touch Homecare LHCSA NY, ASDC, MD's, Nurse Practitioner Groups, FESCO Fire Equipment Company Birmingham/Atlanta/International, Irvin Brother's World Imports, IFPA - International Fire Protection Academy, Hood Master, Southern Fire Solutions, NAFFCO - Dubai, Exit Logic, Jessup Mfg - Chicago, MeridianRx (PBM) - Detroit, and other Healthcare Plans, Providers, Clarity, Tyco, SimplexGrinnell, FireMaster, Clinical, IT, Businesses, Marketing Related Companies, US Military Iraq.

Introduction To No Hogwash Books

This book is not meant to be a masterpiece of grammar. There may be grammatical mistakes. In the spirit of No Hogwash Books, we just try to get straight to the point and to hammer these points home. We are honored that you chose this book to read and study. Some topics in this book may be covered repetitively intentionally.

REMEMBER: It is what you get out of a book that is important. This book is not meant to cover all portions of the subject. It is meant to help you. In order to learn more and grow more we also have courses designed for each subject of interest.

Thanks so much. We are very grateful to consider you a friend.

For more info visit **www.michaelvonirvin.com** Or **www.nohogwashbooks.com**

To work with Michael Von Irvin or make comments contact help@writersprofitguide.com

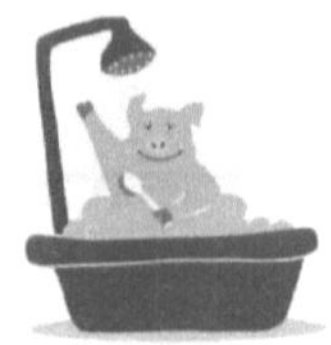

If you are going to make a real change for the better, it will not be easy at first. And know this…..there are a lot of people who are looking out for your best interest. However, there are also a lot of people who will try to control you. I had to break free of negative people and learn how to live my life to the fullest.

-   Michael Von Irvin

Thank you for purchasing this eBook.

Sign up for my FREE eNewsletter and receive special offers, access to bonus content, and info on the latest new releases and other great eBooks from Michael Von Irvin

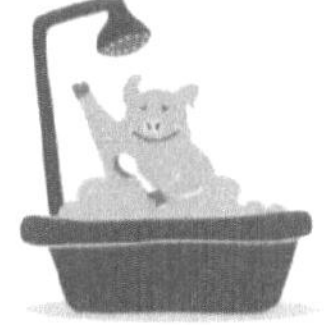

visit us online to sign up
at **www.michaelvonirvin.com**

No Hogwash
De Stress

To work with Michael Von Irvin or make comments contact
help@writersprofitguide.com

The Healthy Way to Get a Handle on Stress

Michael Von Irvin, MBA, BSN, RN

Table of Contents

To work with Michael Von Irvin or make comments contact help@writersprofitguide.com

Conclusion

Disclaimer

Nothing in this book should be construed to be medical advice or even the advice of a nutritionist or dietician. All of the comments herein are from personal experience. The author is absolved from any responsibility regarding any results from those who carry out the suggestions related in this book. Each reader is responsible for his or her own actions.

This and all health related books written by Michael Irvin, RN complement, but do not replace, traditional medical care. This is not to be taken or interpreted as Medical advice. Treatment is your choice. The information here highlights another way to view health and wellness, but it does not diagnose, treat or prescribe; and, it is not intended for primary medical intervention. If you have symptoms, contact your health professional of choice before proceeding with any suggestion book.

Introduction

A woman visited her doctor because she was suffering from blurred vision and continual upset stomach. At one point during the exam the doctor asked the patient, "Are you under any stress?"

She gave a half-hearted laugh and answered, "Of course I'm under stress. Isn't everybody? That's life."

This in a nutshell is our present attitude about stress. It is merely accepted as a part of living life on this planet. While stress may be accepted (a better term might be *endured*), constant stress is eroding the health of an individual quietly and almost unnoticed. When the symptoms begin to manifest (which may be in a multitude of reactions), the sufferer is in a hurry and has little interest in long-term solutions. The answer is nearly always a *quick fix*. This means medication which will then mask the symptoms.

Annually, over $800 million dollars are spent on "anti-anxiety pills." The U.S. accounts for 5% of the world's population and yet they consume 33% of these pills. That's a lot of money to spend on something that is considered by most to be *just a part of living life on this planet.*

Realize that this is just one of many prescription and over-the-counter (OTC) drugs that consumers buy to alleviate a wide array of adverse symptoms causes by excess stress. Many such symptoms are never correctly diagnosed as being related to, or connected with, stress.

Meanwhile the stress continues to grow and build. Sadly, the side effects of many common anti-anxiety and anti-depressant medications are depression and anxiety. (Another way of saying *stress.*) Rather ironic to say the least.

Is stress just a harmless factor that you must learn to accept and live with as a way of life in this crazy, fast-paced, over-scheduled, hurry-to-get-there world? Or is there something within your reach that you can do to cooperate with your body to reduce and diminish the stress in your life – and thereby reduce and diminish the resulting problematic symptoms?

That is what *The Healthy Way to De-Stress* is all about. If you are concerned about your health – both today and in the future – and if you are one who is determined to enjoy optimum health and live life to its fullest, then this book is for you!

Chapter 1

The State of Stress

Stress is Subjective

The problem with stress is that it is so incredibly subjective. What bothers one person (stresses that person), another person doesn't even notice.

"What's that rattle?" (In the car.)

"What rattle? I don't hear any rattle?"

"You don't hear that?"

"No."

"Check the glove compartment. It must be something in there."

"Nope. Nothing rattling there."

"Well, find it! It's driving me nuts!"

Ever experience something like that? The rattle is an irritant to one person, and the other doesn't even hear it. Or at work, one personality grates on the nerves of another personality. Most of the other employees aren't agitated at all.

Two people can go through similar traumatic experiences; one will cope, work through the aftermath, and go on with life. The other is thrown into the depth of despair and suffers years of setbacks.

It's obvious that each person is a unique individual with unique talents, abilities, and personalities. Some tend to be more morose and melancholy, others are more upbeat and optimistic – even when things don't go their way.

Upbringing also plays into how a person reacts to stress. Children who experience highly stressful situations are more prone as adults to accept stress as normal. This might include the death or illness of a parent, an alcoholic parent, and abusive parent, sexual abuse and so on.

On the other hand, the child who grows up in a loving home, who is continually encouraged and affirmed, is more likely to see stress as abnormal. Stress is something to be worked through until it is conquered.

Another factor in stress is the occupation a person chooses. The person who loves their job is apt to rise to the occasion when dealing with stressful events. They see adverse circumstances as welcome challenges.

Not so with the person who hates their job and dreads going to work every day. That person deals with stressful situations differently. Not only do they see adverse circumstances as an everyday occurrence, they feel helpless to do anything about it. They feel a total lack of control.

The current family situation also plays a big part in how a person deals with stress, as well as the stress levels that are present on a daily basis. For instance, if there are serious financial problems in the home, the stress of unpaid bills can become almost unbearable. Again there is the feeling of total loss of control which can grow into chronic depression.

Personality, upbringing, vocation, and family situations are just a few of the wide array of factors that contribute to the levels of stress and how stress is handled in an individual's life.

Stress – Tight

The word *stress* originates from the same Latin word as *strict* which also means *narrow* or *tight*. Stress is said to be caused by forces that limit our freedom and movement.

This definition would indicate outward circumstances and influencers; however, stress actually has two aspects, one that is external and the other that is internal. Life on every hand presents us with disappointments, adverse circumstances, traumatic circumstances, fearful events, obstacles and challenges. The internal aspect of stress is how we react to these reverses in life.

If we become fearful, anxious, angry, bitter, or depressed, such states can lead to a great deal of damage to our health. Internal stress results in the mind always being in an agitated state, the nervous system is thrown off balance, and the immune system is compromised. This then leads to stress-related diseases that are today so prevalent in our society.

While the stress response is necessary in emergency situations, it is unnatural for there to be ongoing stress that is not generated for an emergency. In fact, stress that results from everyday life serves no purpose but to damage our health and disrupt our lives. This happens when we fail to examine the stress and fail to deal with it.

The point is, even though stress appears to be coming at us from all sides, the truth is how we react to the stress – how we deal with the stress – is the determining factor in whether we become the victim of, or the victor over, stress.

Is There a Good Stress?

With all the bad press that stress seems to get these days, it's important to note that not all stress is bad. Think about the muscle tension in all of the muscles in our bodies. If that muscle tension were not there we would collapse in a shapeless mass.

Certain stressors in life keep us active and moving toward our goals. Let's take the person who is a professional public speaker. He is standing backstage ready to step to the microphone. His heart may be pounding and his heart racing. But he welcomes those responses and sees them as the body preparing him for the challenge that lies ahead of him. In other words, this individual is experiencing stress, but he has made the decision to embrace the stress. It is his friend. It is his motivator.

The student who is facing an upcoming exam may be feeling stress, but uses that stress to propel her to be even more diligent about spending time in study and research.

Intense stress can place a person in a *fight or flight* mode which causes the mind to think sharp and clear. Your physical responses are heightened; you become hyper-focused.

Stress can cause stimulation which causes the body to release hormones that boost metabolism. This occurs when chemical signals are sent from the brain's hypothalamus to the pituitary gland to the adrenal cortex. The end of this chain of events is the release of natural steroids such as cortisol and adrenaline.

Cortisol improves your ability to process and use sugars. It allows for faster repair of tissue damage and it shuts down the processes of your body deemed unnecessary at that time, such as digestion.

This could happen to a bride before the wedding just as easily as it can happen to the employee asking the boss for a raise. As you can see none of these reactions are bad; this is good stress. This works well for a short span of time. The problems come when stress is ongoing and ceaseless.

A certain amount of stress is needed just to get up in the morning. It is needed to create strong motivation, and to give you an interest and an excitement about life. Good, or positive, stress, is known as eustress. The difference between positive stress and the negative kind (with which we are more familiar) is the different types of chemicals that are produced in the body. In a *good* stress situation, you get a kind of *runner's high* type of chemical cocktail. Beneficial chemicals like endorphin, serotonin and dopamine are produced and do all sorts of good things for our systems. Interestingly enough, they act rather like antidotes to the bad stress chemicals.

Stress Management

As you continue reading through this book, you will learn more about stress and how it works. You will also learn about stress management which will be the key to unlock the door to overcoming problematic stress. Stress management teaches you how to change from the bad to the good type.

But first let's look at the effects of stress and how important it is to know and understand how these work in your life and in your health.

Chapter 2

The Effects of Stress

Stress is encountered in a wide variety of domains of our lives:

- Relationships

- Social interactions

- Work

- Career

- Finances

- Parenting

- Health

- Planning for the future

- Changes in the environment

- Social upheaval

- Natural and manmade catastrophes

Because it is so prevalent, it's crucial to take a close look at stress. To understand what it is and how it works. As was stated in Chapter 1, for most of us, we just assume stress is a part of life and therefore we are helpless to do much about it. It's just something we have to live with.

Ignoring stress and the subsequent damage it can cause is dangerous to say the least. Again, as long as we minimize the problems of stress we stand to lose a great deal because of it. The many *camouflaged* manifestations of stress is why it's so sinister. In this chapter we'll examine the effects that stress can have and why it should not be ignored. The negative effects of stress are mental and physical and both are equally harmful. We'll look at both areas.

Mental Effects of Excessive Stress

In our days of rushing here and there, striving for possessions, struggling to make ends meet, dealing with relationships that have soured, the joy and peace has drained from our lives. This complex world has robbed us of the everyday pleasures of living fully in the present moment.

Stress is the culprit for preventing us from living in a state of contentment and fulfillment. Think about it. When you are under a great deal of stress, it's impossible for you to feel relaxed and contented. Such emotions simply cannot co-exist.

The greater percentage of stress resides hidden away in the mind area. It seems relatively insignificant. Much of the time it goes unnoticed. It's not until the full-blown physical or behavioral symptoms appear that stress become visible.

Stress can be caused by internal forces such as negative thinking, unrealistic goals, and personal choices (bad habits). These stressors are often due to unrealistic expectations from others and from ourselves; they can also stem from inner conflict and frustration.

The *mind condition* aspect of stress can begin with minor anxiety and slowly develop into depression and from there advance to mental illness. You may read that statement and think this is going to extremes. "After all, it's just a little stress we're talking about."

If only it were that simple. Take a look at these sobering statistics:

- Approximately 50 percent of all admissions to a medical facility are the result of stress.

- Tranquilizers, antidepressants and anti-anxiety medications account for one-fourth of all prescriptions written in the United States each year.

• Anxiety-related disorders account for the highest number of mental illness in this country.

• Major depressive disorders, which include depression, affect an estimated 340 million people worldwide.

• The World Health Organization recently concluded that depression is the world's fourth greatest public health problem.

• Generalized anxiety disorder affects an estimated 183

million people worldwide, the

majority of whom are women.

Add to this list the fact that suicide is the cause of more deaths than homicide or war. The global suicide rate has gone up 60% over the past 45 years. Sixty percent? That's a lot of suicides.

Early symptoms of moderate stress might be such things as:

- Problem sleeping

- Teeth grinding

- Short patience

- Irritability

- Feeling sad

- Anxious

- Lack of ability to concentrate

- Low energy levels

One of the more serious consequences of prolonged stress is the chemical imbalance that happens within the body. There are a number of chemicals in the brain that are known as *neurochemicals*. These are our *feel-good* chemicals that promote a sense of happiness and well being.

The balance of neurochemicals that have been in operation in the human body for millennia has now been disrupted by our modern lives. This disruption causes us to be more prone to depression, anxiety, and malcontent. Sadly, pharmaceutical companies are more than willing to help you to readjust the imbalance with various medications. But these only serve to mask the underlying problem.

Let's look at a few examples of our brain chemicals:

Serotonin

Serotonin is a neurochemical that works to elevate our mood. Stress and anxiety work together to deplete this important neurotransmitter.

Melatonin

Melatonin is primarily responsible for your circadian rhythm, or your biological cycles. When the sun comes up you are awake and feel energized; as it grows dark you begin to feel tired and sleepy. Disrupted melatonin (which can happen through stress) means lethargic tiredness or insomnia.

Dopamine

The neurochemical known as dopamine, which is also produced naturally by your brain, is the *feel good* chemical. You get a rush of dopamine in response to pleasurable activities like food or sex. In the case of low dopamine production, you may feel sluggish, depressed and uninterested in life.

This certainly not an expansive list of the chemicals that your amazing body produces through the brain, but these examples can give you a clearer picture of how and why extended stress can upset your mind and your mental condition. Now we'll take a look at how stress affects our physical bodies.

Physical Effects of Excessive Stress

As was mentioned earlier, in times of trauma and danger, stress causes the human body to go into the *fight or flight* mode. But what happens when the stress is subtle? You are upset, you are aroused physically, but it's inappropriate to respond with the *fight or flight* reaction. What happens now? The body begins to fight against itself.

Digestion

Internalized stress triggers the release of hormones such as adrenaline and cortisol from the adrenal glands. These hormones work to accelerate the pulse rate. Additionally they also activate changes in the digestive system, like lack of appetite, heartburn, nausea, and stomach pains.

Stress can also cause inflammation throughout the digestive system, which leads to irritation of the digestive tract. This irritation will inhibit proper assimilation of nutrients. This means you can eat healthy foods, but if you are overly stressed, your system has difficulty assimilating any nutrition from that food.

Long-term stress will eventually result in chronic digestive problems which could include like irritable bowel syndrome (IBS) and stomach ulcers. Sadly, when a person winds up in the doctor's office complaining of IBS, seldom is stress suggested as the root cause.

Heart

As with the digestive system, prolonged stress negatively affects the heart and the circulatory system. Before the 1920s, heart attacks were fairly rare. Since then things have drastically changed. Now over a million people suffer from heart attacks every year.

At one time it was mostly men over age 65 who experienced heart attacks. Now women also have heart attacks as do those of the younger generation (30s and 40s).

People with what is known as a Type A personality – those who are ambitious, aggressive, competitive and always pushing to be successful – are seven times more apt to suffer a heart attack that those who are live a more laid-back lifestyle. This gives us a glimpse of how excessive stress can play a definite role in heart problems.

The Immune System

Colds, flu, seasonal allergies… Every time something *goes around* you get it. At times you wonder if you're not sick more than you're well. The fact is excessive stress weakens your immune system. The body's immune system is responsible as the front line defense against warring invaders in your body – such as a flu virus.

Rather than dealing with the stress, consumers want the *quick fix.* They head to the drug counter and begin taking the most-popularly advertised product on the shelf that is related to their symptoms.

Or if instead of the drug counter they head to the doctor so they can *get well,* nine times out of ten the prescription is for an antibiotic. Antibiotics are just as their name implies: they are anti – or against – the biotics (bacteria) in the body. The hope is that the antibiotics will rid the body of the problem bacteria. But all the while the antibiotics are killing all of the *good, necessary* bacteria that live in the gut. The first line of defense has now been killed off and the problem will only grow worse.

This becomes a vicious cycle. The stress weakens the immune system; the body become susceptible to infections; the stress increases because the allergies (or whatever the ailment) keep getting worse and the person can't understand why.

Nervous System

Your nervous system is made up of an entire network of nerves (or neurons). All are interconnected and create a massive complex network. The system is made up of two parts:

- The central nervous system (CNS), which includes the brain and the spinal cord

- The peripheral nervous system (PNS), which is a large network of nerves

This amazing system responds to external as well as internal stimuli. The system sends specific instructions to different parts of the body on how to react to a specific stimulus. Do you scream when you see a mouse? Do you jump when startled? Do you faint at the sight of blood? Your neurons are using electrochemical signals to send the messages.

The nervous system is unique in that it not only supervises stress but also controls the body's reactions afterwards. It reduces the level of hormones in the blood stream and signals the heart to revert back to its normal beat rate. This means that following a sudden fright, given time the heart stops pounding, the sweaty palms dry, and the breath evens out. This is the healthy way for the nervous system to function.

Now think about what happens when stress is constant – reverting back to the normal state becomes impossible. This means that the sympathetic nervous system keeps you in a continual state of alert with no let up. This prevents the parasympathetic nervous system from doing its job. Now the body cannot actually rest at all. If the body had no quality rest, the body systems that are suspended during the stress response cannot be resumed effectively.

From this you can clearly see how stress affects every nearly every working part of the systems in your body. And this didn't even touch on the glands such as the lymph glands which are so crucial in cleansing the body and fighting disease.

Stress affects both the mind and body in ways that are greater and more serious than most people ever realize. It's not something we can afford to ignore. It should demand our attention and our resolve to do something about it.

In the next chapter we'll look at what is known as life change units (LCU), and how they affect our stress levels and our lives.

Chapter 3
Life Change Units (LCU)

Cataclysmic Events

In this chapter we'll take a look at the cataclysmic events in life that literally turn our world upside down. Think of those who were affected by the

shooting in the Aurora, Colorado theater on June 20, 2012. Or those who were at the scene at the moment of the Boston Marathon bombing on April 15, 2013. These were ordinary people living ordinary lives going about their ordinary business. They decided to attend a movie. They decided to watch famous Boston Marathon. Suddenly nothing was ordinary any more.

Life changing units (LCUs) can also include surviving a natural disaster like a flood, tornado, or hurricane – such as those who lived through Katrina in 2005. Life changes are much different than what we think of as the daily hassles of daily living. However, they don't have to be as dramatic as a shooting or a bombing.

Other stress-causing life changes can be a move in residence; a child leaving home for the first time; the death of a loved one; a divorce; loss of a job; and the list goes on.

Any of these stressors can be disruptive to our mental and physical health. A study conducted by Stanford University found that after natural disasters, those affected experienced a significant increase in stress level. Further research has shown that those who have been affected by such life changes are much more prone to suffer from a future illness.

Psychologically, a person may suffer from Post Traumatic Stress Disorder (PTSD). One young man who was visiting Israel accidentally stepped on a land mine when he and his friends went for a walk in the countryside. For years he was unable to walk on grass without being terror stricken. He associated the green grass with the moment when his leg was blown off. Such fears and flashbacks are signs of the body reacting to the trauma.

It's not readily understood why some people develop PTSD and others do not. Some individuals experience such events and are able to resume a normal life while others are severely affected for months and even years after.

PTSD sufferers experience difficulty forming, or retaining, close relationships with family and friends. Other symptoms may be lack of trust, inability to be intimate with others, breakdown in communication, and failure in problem solving. The way in which loved ones respond to these problems can further affect the survivor. For instance, those closest to the survivor may distance themselves due to the unnatural behavior.

Holmes and Rahe Stress Scale

In 1967, psychiatrists Thomas Holmes and Richard Rahe did a study of medical records of over 5,000 medical patients as a way to establish if stressful events might indeed result in subsequent illnesses. Patients were required to add up a list of 43 life events based on a relative score. The finding was a positive correlation between their past life events and their current illnesses.

The results of these tests were published as the *Social Readjustment Rating Scale* (SRRS), which later came to be called *the Holmes and Rahe Stress Scale.* Since their initial findings in 1967, subsequent studies have further validated the links between stress and illness.

This test can be found here:

http://www.dartmouth.edu/~eap/library/lifechangestre sstest.pdf

It only takes a few minutes to complete. It will give you a great overview as to where your stress levels might be. For instance if you lost your job, suffered the death of a parent, and then went through a divorce, you might want to take a serious look at preventative measures for your future health. In the upcoming chapters we will look at ways to deal with such traumatic events.

Chapter 4

Daily Stressors

Don't Let it Get To You

The catastrophic events discussed in Chapter 3 are rare and happen only on occasion; however, the daily pressures of life are just that – daily. Most are inescapable.

Have you ever had someone say to you: "Just don't let it get to you." Or the comment might be, "Just don't let her/him get to you." Things *get to us* almost every hour of every day.

While we are told not to let things get to us, or we are told to "just relax," seldom are we told how to do that. In Chapter 1, we established that disappointments, adverse circumstances, traumatic circumstances, fearful events, obstacles and life's challenges can all work as stressors in our daily lives. How these stressors are faced and handled can make a difference in whether or not a person will enjoy a fulfilling, joyful, peaceful life. And whether or not they will achieve their dreams and goals.

Ongoing stress that is ignored or that is masked by drugs and other coping mechanisms can eventually lead to feelings of being *less-than.* This can include feelings of suspiciousness, worthlessness, inadequacy, or rejection. We fear the worst is going to happen and we experience a *case of the nerves* before anything has ever happened. These types of personality changes can be subtle and even if it's pointed out, the person may deny it. We just can't believe we've really changed.

Where do these daily stressors come from? They can be from the nightly news, the latest threat of a layoff at work, dealing with a rebellious teenager, inability to pay bills on time. Some come from our surroundings; others come from our own inner struggles.

Family

Family relationships are multifaceted and oftentimes bewildering. Today the family infrastructure is undergoing tremendous upheaval. Over 40 percent of all children born in this past decade will live in a home with only one parent due to divorce.

Even in families with a strong marriage foundation, there are complex aspects such as the birth of a new baby, aging parents, teens growing up and leaving home, precarious in-law relationships, and so on.

Financial

More and more families find they are living from paycheck to paycheck. Plans they had early on in life are dashed because the finances simply are not there to make them happen. Frustration and hopelessness are mixed with a very real fear – fear of never having enough and fear of their future financial well-being.

Chemical

Many more chemical stressors are in our world today than our grandparents ever experienced. These can be from the water we drink, the air we breathe, the foods we eat, and even the household cleansers we use. Add to this problem the chemicals we knowingly and willingly take into our bodies such as caffeine, nicotine and alcohol.

Change

A few generations ago, a person could live in the same town, work at the same job and be married to the same person for an entire adult lifetime. Change was rare. Not so today. In this day and age change is happening so fast that few if anyone can keep up. Technology has not only changed the way we live, but the way we think. Change is at the same time both expected and yet repulsive.

Today people change jobs and move residences with a great degree of regularity. This means an uprooting, a loss of social networks and support systems. This can be trying for adults, for children, and for adolescents. Individuals who are prone toward depression can be severely affected by such changes.

Additionally, our mindset expects instant results. Sitting through a traffic light two or three times can cause the stomach to be tied in knots. If the garage-door opener fails to work correctly, our teeth grind. So many things throughout the course of the day are affected by the push of one button or another and we expect each one to work instantly. Such a hurried lifestyle adds to the stress levels. We want something *now,* and delays only work to annoy and distress us.

Environmental

Do you have noisy neighbors? Apartment dwellers often have to put up with unwanted noise and disturbances over which they have no control. The same with the workplace. Oftentimes the place where you work may be too noisy or too warm or too cold. Or has insufficient amounts of fresh air. Some people live in an area where pollution is a very real problem and the air quality is an ongoing problem. These environmental problems are areas in which we must endure.

Employment

On-the-job stress has become a common, and a costly problem in the workplace. Statistics show that problems at work are more strongly associated with health complaints than any other stressors – and that includes financial and family problems.

Many employees today are far removed from the end result of their tasks; therefore, it's difficult for them to see the value of their individual contribution. Fewer people today are satisfied with their day-to-day jobs than ever before. Life in a cubicle can have a debilitating effect on some people; they feel caged, confined, unimportant, and undervalued. Such emotions are for the most part tamped down, hidden, and ignored.

The Commute

Getting to and from work is not a problem for every employee, but for those who must spend long hours in backed up traffic, or hours on mass-transit, this can be a valid stressor. Especially after one has already experienced a harrowing work day.

Media

The media majors in bad news – it's an undisputable fact. Bad news sells. All the bad news can come to you via radio, television, computer, the Internet and email. And in today's world, even if you make it a point to avoid all that bad news, you may go into a restaurant, the waiting room of a doctor's office, the waiting room of a car repair shop, or even in the airport terminal, and there it is blaring at you and you have no choice in the matter.

Add to the news the fact that acts of senseless violence are prevalent in the majority of movies and television shows that are produced. These scenes can be so real that our bodies, our minds, and our emotions cannot possibly differentiate the real from the fabricated.

Emotional

Emotional stressors can probably be woven into each of the stressors listed in this section. Our minds are a powerful force and our inner thoughts can become highly destructive. We imagine horrible things are going to happen, or we become convinced that we're going to fail in everything we undertake to do. We feel victimized and helpless by the events swirling all around us. All such negative reactions act as stressors to work against us.

As you look back through this chapter on *Daily Stressors* ask yourself which ones are the most problematic in your daily life. What works to upset you the most? You are probably well aware that this is by no means an exhaustive list, but rather a way to get you to thinking. It's time to be more aware of what *gets to you*, because only then can you begin to take affirmative action and learn how to de-stress your life.

In the next chapter we'll take a look at the most common methods that people use to deal with their overly stressful lives. Which ones fit your life?

Chapter 5

How We Deal With Stress (Conventional Remedies)

Coping Methods

It was mentioned in the previous chapter how we live in an *instant* culture. We want things to happen quickly, and that goes for remedying our problems with stress. We look for the quickest way we can get ourselves calmed down and relaxed. We look for the *quick fix,* and all the while ignore the fact that the stress didn't build in an instant.

What happens when a person feels rattled, or jumpy, or at their wit's end? Most people are way too busy to stop and ascertain exactly what's causing the stress. Or even if they do know (or think they know) the cause of the stress, they have no time to consider ways in which the stress can be *managed.* Instead the great majority of those who are *stressed out* have devised their own set of coping mechanisms.

Coffee

Coffee has become the acceptable drug of choice for millions on a daily basis. Coffee shops are prevalent throughout our nation, and *coffee* breaks at work are not called that by accident. It's safe to say that well over 75% of all coffee drinkers are addicted to the substance. The proof is in the withdrawal reactions if it were suddenly discontinued. While on the surface this consumption seems fairly innocuous a number of problems are hidden from view.

The energy level of a coffee drinker is controlled by the coffee. On any typical day, this person is energized in the morning and lethargic in late afternoon. If morning coffee is not available, there is a notable problem in mental alertness and physical quickness. The person becomes irritable and cannot concentrate. Because our culture so strongly approves of coffee and encourages its use, few coffee drinkers are aware that they are taking a drug.

Caffeine, of course, is not only consumed in the friendly cup of coffee, but also in soda pop. Some types of cola contain even more caffeine than coffee.

Has caffeine become your cure-all for stress? Below are a few questions. If you can answer them correctly, you will get a clearer picture of where caffeine fits into your life.

- Do you drink at least one caffeinated beverage every day?

- Do you experience a headache if you haven't had caffeine at least by mid-day?

- Do you consume at least 4-5 cups of coffees or 3 energy drinks per day?

- Do you experience irritability if you haven't had your morning coffee?

- Does your current caffeine consumption just give you a feeling of normal? (No more boost.)

- Do you spend at least twenty-five dollars per week on coffee or other caffeinated products?

- Do you find yourself planning your day around your caffeine fix?

1. Do you drink more caffeinated beverages than you do plain water?

Honest answers to these questions can give you a better picture of whether or not you do indeed have a caffeine addition.

Tobacco

Another coping mechanism for those under duress is to light up a cigarette. Statistics show that about 19% of all adults over the age of eighteen are smokers. The number is higher for men (21.6%) than for women (16.5%).

The habit of cigarette smoking is as addictive as crack cocaine and even more addictive than heroin. The reason is two-fold:

1.   The pharmacological power of nicotine is one of the strongest stimulants known

2.   The efficiency of smoking as a drug delivery system – the act of smoking puts drugs into the brain more directly than an intravenous injection

Due to its highly harmful effects, cigarette smoking accounts for more than 440,000 deaths (this is one out of every five deaths), in the United States each year. Smoking is the single most preventable cause of major illness, and it is far and away the most serious form of drug abuse in our modern culture.

Thankfully great strides have been made in creating no-smoking areas in work places, restaurants, public transportation, and sporting events. This is commendable since second-hand smoke endangers the health of many non-smokers. Second-hand smoke contains more harmful compounds because it is not filtered through the mat of tobacco.

Smokers experience powerful constrictions of the blood vessels throughout the body. This interferes with blood circulation of the brain and extremities. It raises blood pressure, agitates the digestive system, and irritates the urinary system. The resulting health problems from cigarette smoking are numerous. At the top of the list are respiratory disease and cancer.

In spite of all these problems, still and yet, people light up a cigarette in an effort to calm their nerves. It's a subterfuge at best. It's true that smoking does give a brief interlude of relief of internal tension. But within twenty minutes after that cigarette is crushed out, the tension return stronger than ever. The brain demands another *fix*.

Alcohol

"I'll just grab a quick drink to unwind. It's been a hard day."

Alcohol is yet another in the list of coping mechanisms that stressed out people choose. Similar to cigarette smoking, alcohol is addictive as well as being a powerful health hazard. Also like smoking the release from tension is brief at best and because of its addictive qualities, the body craves more and stronger.

Contrary to the cultural acceptance, alcohol is the strongest and most toxic of the common psychoactive substances. It is actually harder than most of the well-known illegal drugs such as heroin, cocaine and LSD. And yet our society gives out the false impression that it is less dangerous – a falsehood that has been accepted by the public.

The relaxing effects of alcohol can often mask the harmful effects which are highly toxic. Alcohol is poisonous to nerve and liver cells and irritating to the upper digestive tract and urinary system. Additionally, alcohol burns up B-vitamins, especially vitamin B-1 which results in a thiamine deficiency.

As if the contents of plain alcohol were not enough, many beers and wines on the market contain many harmful additives and preservatives which cause further harm to the body.

Comfort Foods

Certain comfort food can be a quick, cheap, and readily available coping mechanism for alleviating stress. These might include greasy fried foods, sweets such as ice cream and candy bars, and salty snacks such as chips and pretzels. Women are much more likely than men to turn to food for stress relief. Such reliance can lead to binge eating and other eating disorders.

Typically it's the person who is feeling a lack of self worth that turns to food to relieve all the *bad* emotions. The food choices in such instances are nearly always high in fats and sugars which tend to be detrimental to one's health.

Such episodes of bingeing, overeating, or continual bad food choices nearly always result in heavy bouts with guilt and self condemnation. Both the eating problem and the condemning thought patterns work to increase stress rather than diminish it.

Tranquilizers and Sedatives

In the ongoing search for a quick fix to our stress problems, many turn to the medical world for help. This often results in a prescription for a tranquilizer or a sedative. Most of these prescription drugs are depressants that interfere with mental function and carry strong risks of addiction.

Billions of dollars are spent each year for stress-relieving drugs and billions of doses of tranquilizers are prescribed each year. If these drugs were working no one would ever need to come back for a second or third prescription. But we all know they are not cures by any sense of the imagination, but are only temporary answers for an ongoing problem.

One of the first effects of prescription sedatives and tranquilizers is a sense of euphoria. Next the normal brain functions are slowed which causes slurred speech, shallow breathing, sluggishness fatigue, disorientation and lack of coordination or dilated pupils. As the body struggles to become accustomed to these drugs the user feels sleepy and uncoordinated. Slowly these symptoms will begin to disappear. Depending on the underlying personality of the individual the drugs can cause one to become agitated or aggressive.

If usage is reduced or stopped, the user may experience withdrawal symptoms, and continued use can lead to physical dependence. Tolerance to the drug's effects can also occur, meaning that larger doses are needed to achieve similar effects as those experienced initially. This may lead users to take higher doses and risk the occurrence of an overdose.

This is not to say that there is never a time or place for prescription drugs in dealing with stress. They are especially effective on a short-term basis following a highly traumatic event such as a death in the family. However, to turn to these substances as an ongoing solution for stress is not only harmful, but futile.

An Experimental Exercise

Looking over this list, you can see what fits your life and your own coping mechanisms. For most people dealing with stress is nothing more than an experimental exercise – over time we develop our own techniques for coping.

- Humor

- Crying

- Talking

- Nervous mannerisms

- Eating

- Alcohol

- Drugs

- Anger

- Withdrawal and mind games

The mind games that people play might include blaming others for our failures, lying or fabricating stories to hide our inadequacies, or slipping into a fantasy world where we lose a sense of reality. The way we cope is largely based on our past experiences. What has helped in the past works as an automatic draw in the present situation. If coffee helped us through the crunch yesterday, we're more likely to grab a cup this morning.

Individual Reactions

The way we learn to cope also has a great deal to do with our own personalities. Some people are *sensitizers* – they are overly sensitive to tension. They are aware of every little change in their body such as a headache, stomachache, or back pain. This then leads to greater stress since it causes worry to arise. On the other hand those who are *repressors* are never aware that they're uptight. Others around them may caution them to slow down but they are oblivious.

This tells us that our reactions to stress can be individualistic and almost automatic. Few of us even think about our reactions to stress. We just deal the best we can and hope it all works out. However, the stresses of our lives tend to increase, and the haphazard approach to handling stress will not end in success.

The sad fact is that hundreds of thousands of people suffer needlessly from physical pain and mental turmoil simply because their coping techniques are not doing the job.

It may surprise you to learn that there is no one magic formula with which to deal with your stress. It's not in a bottle, or in a pill, or in the coffee pot. The good news is there are a number of ways that you can be proactive in 1) learning how to manage your own stress, and 2) learning how to eliminate many stressors in your life.

More about this in the next chapter.

Chapter 6
Natural Stress Relievers

Awareness

In this chapter you will begin to learn more about how to become proactive in the way you deal with stress on a daily basis. You'll be happy to learn that you no longer need to be a victim. It's up to you to become responsible for your life and your health. It's your choice. You can either take control of the stress in your life, or keep on allowing stress to control you.

Much of the answer to becoming proactive is becoming aware. It's time to stop ignoring the stressors; it's time to stop ignoring your stress responses. It's time for a serious self-examination.

Awareness has to do with honesty and living in the present moment. Many of the coping mechanisms listed in the previous chapter do just the opposite. They work to desensitize both the mind and the body. They mask true thoughts and emotions. Slowly over time, the state of *not-feeling* becomes normal, and soon you lose touch with the real *you*. This is not the path to optimum health.

Think back to a time when you were relatively stress free. Recall what it was like to live in a state of contentment. There was no anger or regret of the past, no fear or anxiety about tomorrow. Just a joy of the present moment. You may have to go all the way back to your childhood to remember such a feeling. As you bring these memories to the forefront of your mind – perhaps for the first time in years – it will give you a gauge from which to measure.

Will you ever be able to recreate such a carefree existence? No, of course not. But it is crucial that you bring it to mind and at least have something from which to measure your emotions and state of mind.

After living in a state of denial for a long period of time, it can be difficult to get honest with who you are and where you are in life. Difficult, but not impossible.

Inventory

Are you ready to get serious? You are about to take a vital step toward managing your stress levels. At first it may seem overly simple, but don't underestimate what is explained here. Let's get started.

In a notebook, a journal, or on your computer begin to create an inventory of your life as it has to do with stressors. Begin to list them. All of them. This may take several sessions as they come to your mind. What are the triggers that work to upset you the most? List them. After you have as complete a list as you can possibly create, now ask yourself these questions and write out the answers in your journal:

- How am I adding to the stress in my life?

- What is my main response to stressful situations?

- Are there habit patterns that I can trace?

- What are my thought processes when under stress? (i.e.

hopelessness; anger; vindictiveness; I give up; it's no use)

- What do I like most about my life?
- What do I like least about my life?

By fully and completely answering such thought-provoking questions, you will be forced to be more and more honest with yourself and your present situation. The more honest you become, the more armed you will be in the battle to take back your life.

Sorting and Culling

Once you have a full list created, now it's time to evaluate. You may be surprised to see that some of the items on your list are within your power to change – or to eliminate. For instance, if listening to the nightly news makes your stomach tie up in knots, then turn off the TV before the news comes on. Turn it off and step away.

Your first thought will be, "But I have to keep up with current events." That may be true, but does that mean you have to fill your mind with bad news from around the world (the most of which will never affect you) right before you go to sleep? This is a habit that is easily within your power to break. Create another better habit to take its place, such as listening to soothing music the hour before you retire for the night.

Learn to say No

Another thing that is within your power to change is calendar overload. You may be guilty of saying yes every time someone asks you to do something. You say yes even though you know you have no quality time to give to the task. This may entail a new exercise for you – the ability to say no and mean it.

Many people lack assertiveness for fear of hurting someone's feelings, or for fear of disappointing someone. But this is the time to be honest, remember. If you are asked to do something that you have no heart or desire to do, and you say yes, you are being dishonest. Dishonest with that person and with yourself. This is your life and you are taking control. Try something like this:

> "I feel honored to be invited to be the chairman of the committee. I know it's a worthy cause and a worthy position. However, at this time my plate is full and since I would be unable to commit myself fully I will have to decline. The position deserves someone who can give it their full attention."

Notice the calm and controlled tone of such a response. In some instances you will have to create your own little speech and be prepared by rehearsing it ahead of time. This skill will take time to learn. In some instances you will gain a victory; in other instances you may fall back into your old pattern.

If you have been in the habit of being a yes person for everyone and everything that comes down the pike, it's no wonder you're stressed out. It's time to take back control of your calendar and your schedule.

Cora is a devoted grandma; however she is also a very active grandma. While she loves her grandchildren dearly, she resents the fact that she is called upon to be the babysitter at the most inopportune times. Instead of enjoying the grandchildren, she then becomes angry and feels she was being taken advantage of. (This is also known as the martyr syndrome.) This causes her no end of stress.

Once Cora learned about the techniques of taking control of her life, she set about to create a calendar showing what dates and times she would be available, and placed an X on the dates when she had other plans. She then presented this schedule to all family members involved.

After the initial shock wore off, the family accepted Cora's schedule and respected it. And Cora's own self respect received a big boost. No longer was she placed on the defensive. The stress was alleviated and she was free to have fun with her grandkids.

To work with Michael Von Irvin or make comments contact
help@writersprofitguide.com

Some of the stressors that we complain about the most are well within our power to lessen or be rid of altogether. This is why creating the *stress list* is such an important step in stress management. It had never occurred to Cora that the situation with the grandchildren was such a big stressor in her life. She was so concerned about being a failure as a grandmother that she had allowed others to control her life. Who are you allowing to control your life? How can you make needed changes?

Not All Stressors Can Be Removed

Once you work through your list item by item and remove the stressors that you have control over, now it's time to examine what's left. Obviously not all stressors can ever be removed from your life. And quite honestly, you wouldn't want them to be. Some stressors, as was pointed out earlier in the book, are necessary to live a full, active, and productive life.

For this reason it's counter-productive to treat all stress the same. A cup of coffee does that. As does a cigarette and a tranquilizer. None of these so-called stress relievers are able to discern between good stress and bad stress. Furthermore, by treating all stress with one or two of your favorite stress relievers, your mind and emotions will never learn how to process or cope. In other words, you will never learn effective stress management by masking the stress itself.

In Chapter 2, the various chemicals in the brain were discussed. The first step in stress management is to cooperate with these chemicals rather than suppress them. Tobacco, caffeine, poor eating habits, and prescription drugs all work to suppress these beneficial chemicals. Is it any wonder that we struggle with high stress levels?

Sleep and Rest

In generations past, most especially in an agrarian culture, daily schedules were ruled naturally by the rising and setting of the sun. This natural balance is called the circadian rhythms. The natural rhythm for the hormone cortisol is for it to be secreted in the morning in relatively high levels to boost the body into action. Lower levels of cortisol are secreted at night which naturally allows the body to prepare for sleep and rest. Because we now have sufficient artificial light twenty-four hours a day, it's easy to stay up into the late hours and then suffer from sleep deprivation the following day.

Check your *stress list* to see if you have listed *overwork* as one of your stressors. If you are pushing yourself too hard, you may not be getting enough sleep, or you are not getting quality sleep. Believe it, the quality of your sleep directly affects the quality of your waking life. This involves your mental state of well being, your emotional balance, and even your physical energy.

The Type A personality was mentioned in Chapter 2. This personality is especially prone to push their body past its normal endurance, and this includes lack of sleep. It is almost like a badge of honor to be able to go at a fast pace with very little sleep, never fully realizing the toll it takes on their health. Sooner or later the damage will begin to manifest.

Some of the more common effects of sleep deprivation is elevated blood pressure and weakened immune system. We also know that lack of sleep hinders the body from being able to manage stress. Conversely heightened stress affects quality of sleep; thus it becomes a vicious cycle. But it's a cycle that can be broken.

Now that you have become aware, now that you are ready to take control of your life, it's time to take action. Create your own personal routine to achieve quality sleep. This will definitely include setting a time by which you will go to bed. The only exceptions will be in cases of emergencies. Here are a few other wind-down ideas:

- Say no to any commitments that rob your personal evening time
- Avoid serious meetings or discussions before going to bed
- Avoid strenuous exercise just before bedtime
- Avoid any type of caffeine during the evening hours
- Reserve the bedroom for relaxing, reflecting, loving and sleeping (no exceptions)
- Listen to soft, soothing music during the evening hours
- Have the room dark and quiet (a face mask may be needed to ensure suitable darkness)
- Take a hot bath twenty minutes before bedtime (add Epsom salts or your favorite relaxing oils such as lavender)

Taking these steps can, quite literally, change your life. It's difficult to fully appreciate how important sleep is to your overall health until it is restored and you begin to feel the life-giving effects.

Physical Exercise

People who discover what an amazing stress reliever physical exercise rarely spend money on sedatives or tranquilizers. If you haven't yet caught hold of this extremely effective, and yet incredibly inexpensive, stress management technique, the time is now.

No more excuses about how you don't like to exercise, or don't have time. The changes that can happen in your physical and emotional health are nothing short of magical. Our bodies were created to be in motion. (Actually that is a good kind of stress.) Find something you like – something you very much enjoy doing. Your exercise program doesn't have to be a membership at the local health club or spa. It can start with an after-supper walk around the block.

If you have not been exercising up until now, start out slow and work up until you have developed a well-established habit pattern. Some people love the gym or health club, especially the community atmosphere. Others like jogging outside in the fresh air. Still others like their exercise DVDs where they can work out in front of the TV in their own living room. Don't rule out biking or swimming. The more you enjoy the particular exercise – and the place where you exercise – the more apt you are to maintain. And maintenance is crucial. Creating your own personal exercise routine will be a change in lifestyle, far removed from a quick-fix pill.

Deep Muscle Relaxation

Yet another stress management technique is deep muscle relaxation (also known as progressive muscle relaxation). This exercise involves a two-step process. The first step is to systematically tense a set of muscle groups in your body (this could be your neck and shoulders which is notorious for holding stress). After tensing these muscles and holding it for a few seconds, you release the tension. Now take notice of how your muscles feel when they are relaxed.

This is such a simple exercise and yet holds powerful benefits. Through this method you can quickly and effectively lower your overall tension and stress levels. Use this to relieve anxious feelings instead of grabbing that extra cup of coffee.

The best way to learn this technique is to set aside fifteen minutes or so and retire to a quiet room where you can sit comfortably and not be disturbed. A recliner works well, or a comfortable armchair. A bed is not advised because this is not to put you to sleep; it's to teach you relaxing methods when awake. Be sure to wear loose clothing.

To work with Michael Von Irvin or make comments contact
help@writersprofitguide.com

Begin walking through this process twice a day until you learn exactly how it's done. Don't wait until you are anxious to begin your learning sessions – start when you are calm. This learning process will then stand you in good stead when you do become anxious and upset.

Start with one muscle group such as your left hand. Make a tight fist and hold it for a few seconds. Now release. As you release exhale and pay attention to how the muscles feel as they go free and limp. Think of the tension flowing out and away from you. The most important part of the whole exercise is that you deliberately focus on the different feeling between tense and relaxed muscles. Only concentrate on one muscle group at a time. This is why you need at least fifteen minutes to complete. You want to cover the entire body.

Once you have conquered the areas of quality sleep, exercise, and deep muscle relaxation, you will be way down the road in the area of stress management. But this is still not a total answer. Let's look at how you can cooperate with your mind.

Mental Stress Management

No one needs to tell you that ongoing stress, fear, and panic are destructive habit patterns. One of the mental stress management skills is to stop for a moment and reflect. Purposely change the course of your thought patterns. If your mind is whirling with negative and anxious thoughts it's time to put meditation into practice. As with learning deep muscle relaxation, meditation will take time to learn and perfect.

Meditation involves focusing your mind on a single object. Your main goal is to slow the thoughts that are spinning in your head. They are bouncing here and there but they are getting you nowhere. They are in no way constructive, but only destructive.

Choose that one object on which to concentrate. It can be a visible object that you look at, or it can be something like your very own breath. Because you cannot think about two different things at one time, the wild distracting thoughts will dissipate; your mind will grow quiet. After a few moments of meditation you are now fully in the present.

To work with Michael Von Irvin or make comments contact
help@writersprofitguide.com

If the negative thoughts try to come back in, do not get upset at yourself or at the thoughts. Slowly and patiently bring the thoughts back to the center of concentration.

Be aware this is not easy to achieve at first. Why? Because your mind has been so used to darting about wherever it pleases so it will continue to try to go its own way. You remain in quiet control. Consistently you rein the thoughts back in and remain focused.

Begin with only a few minutes at a time, and slowly increase with each session. Soon you will be so adept at meditation, you will move into that quiet mode in your most anxious moments no matter where you are.

It has been proven that habitual meditation as described here, increases memory and concentration. Tension, anxiety and frustration fade away. When those loud, demanding thoughts inside your head are stilled, you will experience a sense of inner peace and well-being.

Visualization

Another mental exercise that is used by elite athletes to stay on top of their game is that of visualization. *Visualize to actualize* as the saying goes. Begin to see yourself as a relaxed, in-charge person. One who achieves goals, who lives life to the fullest, enjoys optimum health, and daily enjoys peace of mind and a state of well being.

Some people use vision boards where pictures are posted that depict these lifestyle achievements. Having the pictures to look at each day brings a sense of realism to the visualization. The realism makes the achievement seem even more probable and possible.

This chapter has presented only a few of the many natural remedies for managing daily stress. There are so many more such as biofeedback, yoga, imagery that involves the five senses, and even martial arts. Hopefully what has been introduced here will give you a clearer picture of your power of control. Ignoring stress, seeing it as something must be endured, or treating it with destructive habits such as caffeine or nicotine, will never be the full answer.

To work with Michael Von Irvin or make comments contact
help@writersprofitguide.com

In the final chapter we'll look at how what you eat affects your stress levels.

Chapter 7 Stress and Nutrition

Far From the Hippocratic Oath

Many of the so-called stress relievers do nothing for long-term stress reduction. As we saw in Chapter 2, most work just the opposite. Not only do they not reduce stress, they produce a strong rebound effect which means more and more is needed just to achieve a feeling of normalcy. This makes them highly addictive. The alternative is a healthy diet which works to cooperate with all of the natural stress relievers that the body has to offer.

Much of what Americans consume these days is not food at all but a chemical derivative of what was once a nutritious food product. Processed foods not only remove precious nutrients that our bodies require for optimum health, but they contain harmful chemical additives many of which our bodies do not even recognize. This in turn taxes vital organs such as the heart, lungs, liver, and stomach, not to mention the immune system.

How far we've come since Hippocrates, the Greek father of modern medicine who stated over 2000 years ago: *Let food be your medicine and medicine be your food.* Even he understood that it matters what we eat, and that was long before processed foods came into being. It's important that the foods you eat are foods that support a healthy neurochemical balance.

If you are determined to cooperate with your natural stress resistors, if you want a body that is geared to effectively deal with stress, then be prepared to make a few lifestyle changes – and it can begin in your own kitchen.

As was mentioned regarding prescription and over-the-counter drugs that are taken for stress reduction, processed foods also work against the body's natural stress relievers. A person who is under a great deal of stress further exacerbates the problem by ingesting foods that lack the needed vitamins and minerals requisite for optimum health.

The natural stress relievers outlined in the previous chapter are all easy to implement and are relatively low-cost. The same can be said for changing to a healthy diet.

What's In Your Pantry?

One of the most basic methods of changing over to a healthy diet is to consume foods that are as near to their natural state as is possible. Eat a real carrot; a real head of broccoli; a real green bean; a real squash. Take inventory of your kitchen to see what is packaged and therefore low in nutrients. As you see with a new set of eyes (you're serious about conquering the stress problem remember), look for items that can be exchanged.

Don't attempt to make drastic changes all at once – such actions seldom work. Be purposeful, strategic, thorough, and practical. As you run out of a packaged food item, simply refuse to re-stock it. Meanwhile shop the perimeter of the grocery store. This is where you find the *live food items*. It's in the center aisles where all the packaged food items are stored.

As you learn to cook and eat healthy, you can set up your own exchange system. Exchange white flour for whole grain; exchange white flour bread items for whole grain bread items; exchange refined sugar for natural sweeteners (honey, stevia, agave nectar, blackstrap molasses, and barley malt syrup); exchange sweet soda pop for plain water or water with fresh lemon; exchange coffee for herbal tea. And the list goes on and on.

Juicing fresh fruits and vegetables is a quick and easy way to infuse your body with added vitamins and minerals. Those who establish a habit of juicing first thing in the morning find that their caffeine cravings soon disappear. That false boost is no longer needed.

As you slowly eliminate the harmful and non-nutritious food items from your diet, you will begin to experience higher energy levels. Your thinking will be clear and your level of concentration will increase. It is the healthy mind and body that is able to diffuse the anxious moments in life. It is the healthy mind and body that is able to deal with unavoidable stressors in life.

It doesn't take much research for you to learn what foods are good for you and which ones are not. If you have never heard of the glycemic index it will be of great benefit to be informed. High-GI foods are linked to diseases such as diabetes and heart disease. Low-GI foods are high in nutrition and give sustained energy. Learn more at this website: http://www.glycemicindex.com/

The more you educate yourself in the areas of nutrition and wellness the more in control of your life you will be. And, in turn, the more in control you will be with regards to stress management.

Conclusion

Which do your prefer? To be controlled by the ongoing stress and stressors in your life? Or to be in control of your mind, your will, your health, and your emotions? Hopefully, you have chosen the latter. No longer do you need to say like the lady mentioned in the introduction: "Of course I'm under stress. Isn't everybody? That's life."

Never again will you ignore the stress; never again will you feel the need to use quick-fix remedies that cannot ever affect a permanent cure. You are serious; you are determined; you are purpose-filled. You want your life to count; you want to be in control; you want to be the victor over excessive stress and not the victim.

To work with Michael Von Irvin or make comments contact
help@writersprofitguide.com

You will never come to terms with the stress in your life by trying to disown it ("Oh, it's nothing. Just something I have to live with.") or suppress it ("I'm fine just as long as I have a few downers and a cup of coffee."). The only way to be in control of your stress-filled life is to own every facet of the stress – acknowledge them, understand them, and recognize which can be eliminated and which need to be carefully managed. Only then will you be able to constructively use all your energy to enjoy optimum health, peace of mind, and live in a state of well being every day of your life.

Here's to your healthy, stress-overcoming life.

Control Stress Before It Causes You or Others Harm Or Worse Learn Techniques and Tips For The Healthy Way To Deal With Your Stress And Enjoy Life De Stress Your Life

To work with Michael Von Irvin or make comments contact
help@writersprofitguide.com

Michael Irvin is an internationally recognized as health expert, marketing expert, businessman, and author who has helped others earn millions of dollars. He has helped people in just about every business category turn their ideas into fortunes. Michael's Limitless Health approach is straight forward and aims to cut through the hype found in typical business and health related world. His advice has been given and accepted by successful people throughout the world. He wrote the Limitless Health Series in order to give straight forward information without the hype. For more money making and marketing tips and techniques, tactics, and strategies, go to michaelvonirvin.com

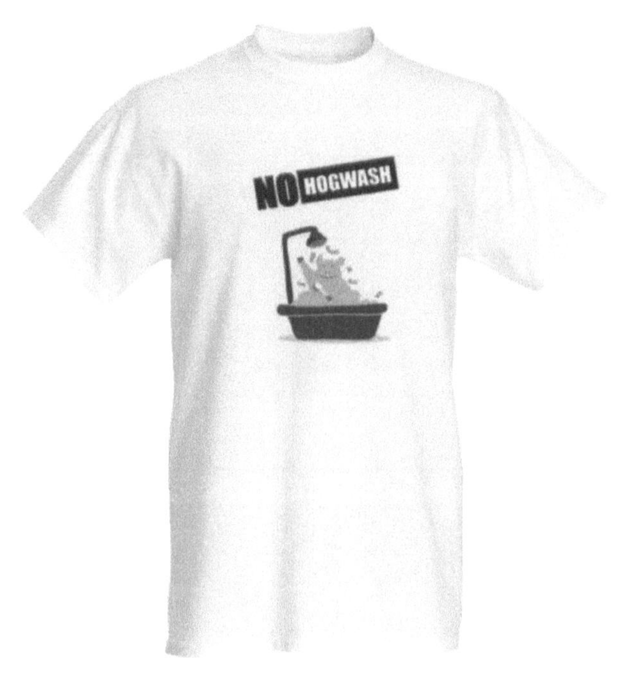

To work with Michael Von Irvin or make comments contact
help@writersprofitguide.com

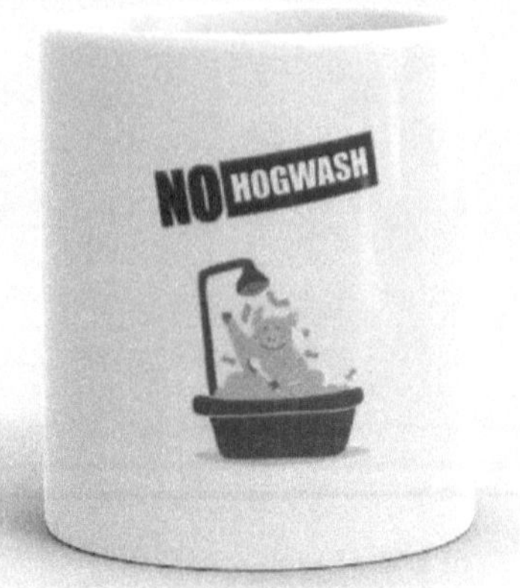

NO HOGWASH

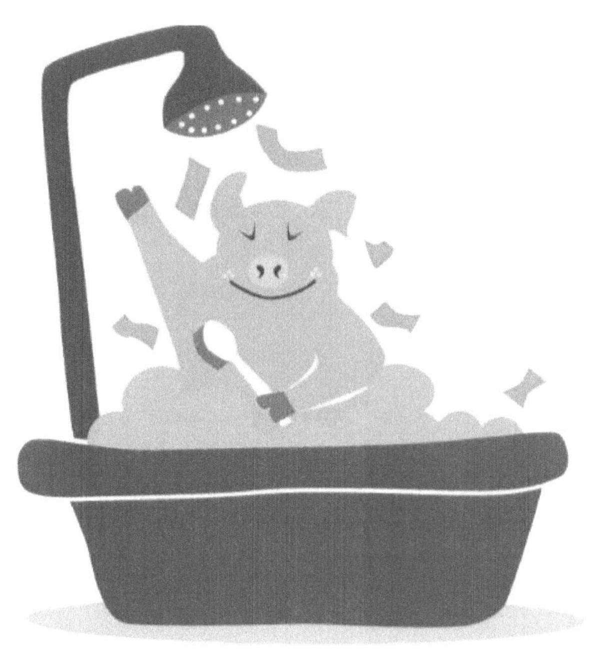

To work with Michael Von Irvin or make comments contact
help@writersprofitguide.com

NO HOGWASH

9 781794 499638